YOUR KNOWLEDGE HAS VALUE

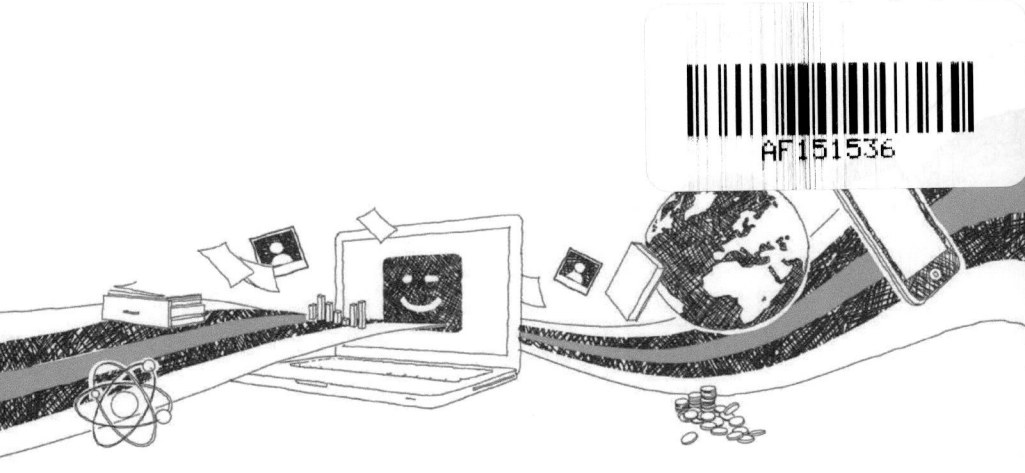
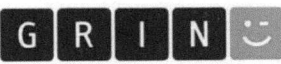

Hossam Hassan Khamis, Azza Galal Farghaly, Hanan Zakaria Shatat, Engy Mohamed El-Ghitany

Prevalence of hepatitis C virus infection among pregnant women in a rural district in Egypt

GRIN Publishing

Bibliographic information published by the German National Library:

The German National Library lists this publication in the National Bibliography; detailed bibliographic data are available on the Internet at http://dnb.dnb.de .

Imprint:

Copyright © 2015 GRIN Verlag GmbH
Print and binding: Books on Demand GmbH, Norderstedt Germany
ISBN: 978-3-656-91658-1

This book at GRIN:

http://www.grin.com/en/e-book/293845/prevalence-of-hepatitis-c-virus-infection-among-pregnant-women-in-a-rural

GRIN - Your knowledge has value

Since its foundation in 1998, GRIN has specialized in publishing academic texts by students, college teachers and other academics as e-book and printed book. The website www.grin.com is an ideal platform for presenting term papers, final papers, scientific essays, dissertations and specialist books.

Visit us on the internet:

http://www.grin.com/

http://www.facebook.com/grincom

http://www.twitter.com/grin_com

Prevalence of hepatitis C virus infection among pregnant women in a rural district in Egypt.

HCV in Egyptian rural pregnant woman.

By Dr. Hossam Hassan Khamis

Supervision committee:

1. **Prof. Dr. Azza Galal Farghaly**
   Professor of Tropical Health
   Department of Tropical Health
   High Institute of Public Health
   University of Alexandria

2. **Prof. Dr. Hanan Zakaria Shatat**
   Professor of Tropical Health
   Department of Tropical Health
   High Institute of Public Health
   University of Alexandria

3. **Assistant Prof. Dr. Engy Mohamed El-Ghitany**
   Assistant Professor of Tropical Health
   Department of Tropical Health
   High Institute of Public Health
   University of Alexandria

"This book is dedicated to my brilliant wife without whom I would be nothing. She always comforts and consoles, never complains or interferes, asks nothing, and endures all.

Hossam Khamis

THE AUTHORS

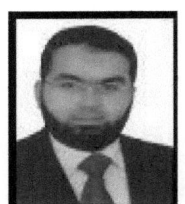**Dr. Hosaam Hassan Khamis** is the corresponding author of this research, he is a tropical medicine resident doctor in Alexandria fevers hospital.

This research was submitted in partial fulfillment of the requirements for the master degree of public health from the high institute of public health in Alexandria university, Egypt.

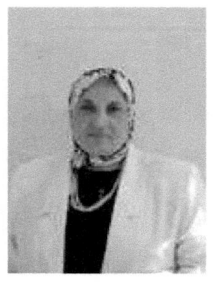

Prof. Dr. Azza Galal Farghaly, Professor of Tropical Health ,Department of Tropical Health ,High Institute of Public Health,University of Alexandria.

She participated in this research by supervising the laboratory diagnosis of HCV seropositivity using ELISA technique, and She also helped the student in interpreting results and revising the thesis.

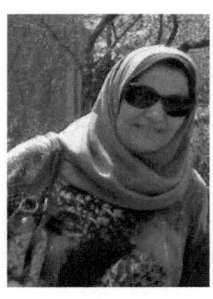 **Prof. Dr. Hanan Zakaria Shatat,** Professor of Tropical Health , Department of Tropical Health ,High Institute of Public Health,University of Alexandria.

She participated in this research by helping the student in data interpretation and revising all thesis sections.

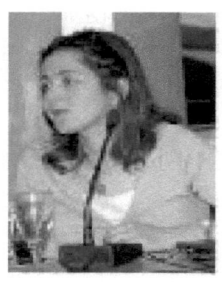

Assistant Prof. Dr. Engy Mohamed El-Ghitany, Department of Tropical Health, High Institute of Public Health, University of Alexandria.

She supervised the student in preparation of questionnaire form and she guided him in interpreting and presenting the results and revising all sections of thesis.

LIST OF CONTENTS

Chapter	Page

LIST OF TABLES

LIST OF FIGURES

INTRODUCTION

INTRODUCTION

Epidemiology:

It is estimated that 130–170 million people, or approximately 3% of the world's population, are living with chronic hepatitis C. About 3–4 million people are infected per year, and more than 350,000 people die yearly from hepatitis C-related diseases.[1] Rates have increased substantially in the 20th century due to intravenous drug use, intravenous medication and poorly sterilized medical equipment.[2]

With 75–85% rate of chronicity ,[2] cirrhosis develops in around 10% of chronic cases in 20 years and the percentage increases to 20% in 30 years. The annual rate of mortality in cirrhotic patients is approximatly 1–5% per year and that of hepatocellular carcinoma is 12.8 % per year. Among those chronically infected, the risk of cirrhosis after 20 years varies between studies but has been estimated at approximately 10-15% for men and approximately 1-5% for women. The reason for this difference is not known. [3]

In the United States, about 2% of people have hepatitis C with about 35,000 to 185,000 new cases a year. Rates have decreased in the Western world since the 1990s due to improved screening of blood before transfusion and infection control measures. Annual deaths from HCV in the United States range from 8,000 to 10,000.Expectations are that this mortality rate will increase, as those infected by transfusion before HCV testing become apparent. [4]

Prevalence is higher in some countries in Africa and Asia.[5]Countries with particularly high rates of infection include Egypt (22%), Pakistan (4.8%) and China (3.2%) .[6]

HCV in Egypt:

A recent study has been made about HCV in Egypt and had found that the incidence was about 7/1000 rate with prevalence of 14.7%. One in every 10 Egyptians is a carrier of the HCV infection, which means that there are at least 4,459,000 persons infected with HCV who are infectious to others. This is the largest reservoir of HCV infection in the world. The study estimates that more than 500,000 new HCV infections occur in Egypt every year, likely signalling an epidemic in a country of more than 85 million people. The authors suggest that this high rate of HCV transmission may be due to the lack of sufficient standard safety precautions in medical and dental facilities. Although the high prevalence of hepatitis C in Egypt has been well established for many years, and linked in part to limited safety measures during anti-bilharzia campaigns, published estimates of prevalence from different Egyptian communities failed to provide a nationwide picture of the magnitude of ongoing HCV infection transmission.[7]

Modes of transmission and risk factors:

Case-control studies before 1989 of patients with newly acquired, symptomatic non-A, non-B hepatitis found a significant association between disease acquisition and a six-months prior to illness history of blood transfusions, injection drug use, health care employment with frequent exposure to blood, personal contact with others who had hepatitis, multiple sexual partners or low socioeconomic status.[8]

Blood transfusion/receipt of blood products :

Today, HCV is rarely transmitted by blood transfusion or transplantation of organs due to thorough screening of the blood supply for the presence of the virus and inactivation procedures that destroy blood borne viruses. In the last several years, some blood banks have instituted techniques that utilize nucleic acid amplification of the hepatitis C virus (NAT), which will detect the presence of virus even in newly-infected patients who are still hepatitis C antibody-negative. These techniques are estimated to have prevented 56 transfusion-associated HCV infections per year in the U.S. since 1999, and have lowered the current risk of acquiring HCV via transfused blood products to 1 in 2 million.[9]Although NAT is very beneficial as it becomes positive more quickly and remains positive as long as the virus is present but it is very expensive in developing countries so other much cheaper tests like ELISA can be used as it has objective results , much lower cost, and appreciable sensitivity(99.7%) [10]

Injection drug use:

Injection drug (IDU) use has been the principal mode of transmission of HCV since the 1970's.[11]Rates of HCV infection among young IDU are four times higher than HIV infection.[12]Studies of IDU have demonstrated that the prevalence of HCV infection in them is extremely high, with up to 90% having been exposed.[13]In addition, the incidence of new infections is also high, with seroconversion rates of 10-20 percent per year.[14]Duration of being IDU is the strongest single predictor of risk of HCV infection among them.[15]

Sexual transmission:

Sexual transmission of HCV has been controversial. It is believed that HCV can be transmitted sexually, but that such transmission is inefficient. The likelihood of HCV infection increases with the number of lifetime sexual partners. A history of a sexually transmitted disease, sex with a prostitute, more than five sexual partners per year, or a combination of these has been independently associated with positive HCV serology.[16]Distinction appears to exist between the specific sexual behaviors listed above, and stable, monogamous sexual activity, which is rarely associated with HCV transmission. The frequency of HCV transmission between monogamous sexual partners is very low according to most published studies.[17,18]

Prenatal transmission:

Although mother to infant transmission of HCV is comparatively uncommon, it is the major route of infection to infants. Transmission may occur during pregnancy, delivery or postnatally through breastfeeding or other contact methods. Infants who are born to HCV Ab positive mothers found to have (81%) seropositivity for HCV antibody at the first month, but only (13%) were positive for HCV RNA. After 6 months, only (3.8%) remained positive for HCV RNA. The chance of infection is greater (17%) with higher serum level of HCV RNA (above 10^6 copies per mL) and in mothers co-infected with HIV (14%).[19]

Other modes of transmission:

Household transmission:

In Egypt the strongest predictor of incident HCV was having an anti-HCV-positive family member. Among those who have HCV positive family member incidence was 5.8/1,000 per year, compared with 1.0/1,000 per year among those who have not.[20] Although the prevalence of HCV among household contacts of people with HCV infection is detectable the study of HCV transmission among household contacts is complicated by the difficulty in ruling out other possible modes of acquisition. Therefore, other routes of transmission might be under estimated. [21]

Occupational exposures:

Health care workers who have exposure to blood are at risk of infection with HCV and other bloodborne pathogens. The prevalence of HCV infection, however, is not greater in health care workers, including surgeons, than for the general population. According to the Centers for Disease Control and Prevention (CDC), the average rate of anti-HCV seroconversion after unintentional needlesticks or sharps exposure from an HCV-positive source is 1.8% (range 0%-7%). An Italian study of 4,403 needlestick exposure among healthcare workers only 14(0.31%) seroconversions were reported.[22] Close follow-up of health care workers after a needlestick from a patient with chronic HCV, with early interferon and ribavirin therapy for the healthcare worker if they develop HCV viremia can be a beneficial management strategy.[23]

No Identifiable Source of Infection:

According to the CDC, injection drug use accounts for approximately 60% of all HCV infections, while other known exposures account for 20-30%.[12]Approximately 10-12% of patients in most epidemiological studies, however, have no identifiable source of infection.HCV exposure in these patients may be from a number of uncommon modes of transmission, including vertical transmission, and parenteral transmission from medical or dental procedures prior to the availability of HCV testing. There are no conclusive data to show that persons with a history of exposures such as intranasal cocaine use, tattooing or body piercing are at an increased risk for HCV infection based on these exposures solely. It is believed, however, that these are potential modes of HCV acquisition in the absence of adequate sterilization techniques.[24]

HCV and pregnancy:

Estimates of the prevalence of HCV infection in pregnant women vary widely among studies, ranging from 0.1% to 4.5% worldwide but in Egypt it was estimated to be about 10.8%.[25] The presence of HCV infection does not appear to result in a higher risk pregnancy or a higher incidence of poor obstetric outcome. [26]

The rate of vertical transmission of HCV has also been estimated with widely varying results. The difficulty of obtaining accurate measurement of vertical transmission risk includes persistence of maternal antibodies in the newborn, failure to identify all infected mothers and loss of infants born to HCV positive mothers to follow-up. The prevalence of vertical transmission of HCV is in the range of 5%. Although HCV/ HIV co-infection appears to increase the risk of vertical transmission, other risk factors have not been consistently identified. Even the identification of the timing of such transmission between intrauterine versus intrapartum exposure has not been satisfactorily delineated. It is not clear that high viral load or viral genotype increases the risk of transmission.[26]

Testing for the presence of HCV in infants born to HCV(+) mothers should not begin until at least 18 months following delivery.[20]

Prophylactic caesarian section is not recommended in HCV infected or HCV/HIV coinfected mothers. In cases of labor with prolonged rupture of membranes, the increased risk of HCV transmission may affect the decision for operative delivery. The risk of postnatal transmission through breastfeeding or any other contact methods cannot be excluded but is likely to be low for most HCV-infected women.[26]

Pregnancy, however, may be an important time to screen for HCV infection. Many women will already have reached their peak likelihood of becoming infected by the time they become pregnant, making the yield of testing near its maximum. Screening at this point in a woman's life can also provide early diagnosis and treatment that may offset the future burden of HCV on the health care system. Further, testing for HCV during pregnancy may help to identify infected newborns, allowing for appropriate follow-up.

HCV in children:

The natural history of HCV infected infants is poorly understood at this time. HCV is the most common cause of chronic liver disease of infectious etiology in children. In a research which is made among school children in Alexandria, HCV seroprevalence of 5.8% was found, with HCV viraemia in 75% of the studied children. The prevalence of anti-HCV increased with age from 0% in children aged 6-7 years to 16% in those of 15 years old. [27]

Previous blood transfusion ,intravenous injections, surgical intervention, dental treatment, circumcision for boys by informal health care providers, age above 10 years ,very low socioeconomic class and rural area residence are the most significant risk factors for HCV infection in children.[28]

Globally, while the number of new HCV infections in adults is declining, new infections in children continue to occur as a result of maternal-neonatal transmission. A sizeable number of children acquired HCV via blood and blood products. Vertical transmission, or infection transmitted from mother to newborn, accounts for another sizeable group of children with HCV infection. Horizontal transmission, either from adult to child in a household, or child-to-child at home or at school does not seem to be an important risk factor. [28]

Acute HCV infection in children is rarely observed unless there are special circumstances such as a transfusion-associated outbreak. Fulminant hepatic failure from HCV has not been described in children. [28]

Most chronically infected children with HCV are asymptomatic (without complaints) or have non-specific fatigue and/or abdominal pain. Most children with HCV infection have normal or mildly abnormal serum transaminase levels. Natural history studies in children are few, and it is difficult to separate the effects of age and mode of acquisition. Further, depending upon the underlying disease that required a transfusion, the natural history of transfusion-associated HCV infection may differ. [28]

There are no reports of treatment of acute HCV infection in children. A review of the use of interferon as monotherapy in children demonstrates a sustained virologic response (SVR) of 33-45%. This is significantly better then the sustained virologic response rate for interferon monotherapy observed for adults. When the data is further scrutinized, the SVR for genotype 1 is 26% and 70% for genotypes 2 and 3. The higher response rate observed in children might be the result of the earlier stage of the disease, higher relative interferon dosage, or lack of comorbid conditions Side effects can be seen as mild symptoms e.g: nausea, vomiting, heartburn, loss of appetite, changes in taste, dry mouth, dry cough, diarrhea, or severe as chest pain, heart attack, congestive heart failure, stroke, low or high blood pressure, decrease in kidney function and failure, jaundice and changes in vision. The experiences with therapy in children with chronic hepatitis C are based on earlier and continuing data from adult trials.Further researches are so much needed to provide the scientific tools to prevent and treat HCV infection in children. [29]

Preventive measures:

The principle components of the National CDC HCV Prevention Strategy are: [30]

• **Primary prevention activities include:**

- Screening and testing of blood, plasma, organ, tissue, and semen donors.
- Virus inactivation of plasma-derived products.
- Adequate sterilization of reusable material such as surgical or dental instruments.
- Risk-reduction counseling and services.
- Implementation and maintenance of infection-control practices
- Needle and syringe exchange programs

• **Secondary prevention activities include:**

- Identification, counseling, and testing of persons at risk
- Medical management of infected persons
- Professional and public education
- Surveillance and research to monitor disease trends and the effectiveness of prevention activities and to develop improved prevention methods.
- Prevention of spread of infection should be the main goal at the current time until cost effective therapies become available.

AIM OF THE STUDY

AIM OF THE STUDY

General objective:

To study the prevalence of HCV infection among pregnant women in Al-Nobareya town, Al-Beheira Governorate.

Specific objectives:

1- To estimate anti-HCV seropositivity rate among pregnant women in Al-Nobareya town, Al-Beheira Governorate.

2- To identify risk factors of HCV infection among pregnant women in Al-Nobareya town, Al-Beheira Governorate.

PLAN OF THE STUDY

PLAN OF THE STUDY

Study setting:

There are 14 villages affiliated to Al-nobareya town, most of residents of these villages were moving recently from different rural governorates to live and work in that new villages. The total population size is 60588 persons according to Al-beheira Governorate. (personal communication with Elbeheira Governorate).

We randomly selected 9 villages namely; Belal, Abo elyosr, Elishaa, Soliman, Adam, Abd Elwahab, Abd Alrakeeb, Alemam Malek and Yousef..

Each one of the selected villages is designed to be one kilometer square and their population sizes are 6120 ,4209 ,6125 ,4143 ,6360 ,4550, 5540, 6790,5370 respectively representing about half the total population of Al-nobareya town.

Each of the selected village has one antenatal health care unit. This study was carried out among pregnant women visiting the antenatal health care units in the selected villages.

Study design:

Cross-sectional study.

Study population:

Inclusion criteria:

Pregnant women attending the study setting for routine antenatal care regardless of gestational age.

11

Exclusion criteria:

- Pregnant women known to be HCV infected.

- History of chronic liver disease.

Sampling design:

Sample size:

Using a power of 80 %, an alpha error of 0.05 and a precision of 2%, the minimal required sample size to estimate the prevalence of HCV infection among pregnant women was found to be 360 cases. The sample size was calculated using STATA software and depending on a prevalence of 10.8 %.[25]

Sampling:

For nearly 18 weeks one of the participating antenatal health care units was visited each week and sometimes the researcher had to visit the same unit more than once. The purpose was to include all eligible pregnant women visiting these units. The participating women had to give an informed consent before enrolment in the study. Each visit about 20 women were included. All the included women underwent the following:

Data collection method:

A. A pre designed questionnaire was filled. It contained data regarding socio-demographic and contact data (name, age, occupation, education, address, telephone number) and data regarding possible risk factors (history of operation, dental procedure, blood transfusion, tattooing, circumcision, intravenous drugs, invasive procedures, HCV +ve husband, family history, etc).

B- Laboratory tests:

A five ml blood sample was withdrawn using the universal sterile precautions. Each visit 20-30 samples were obtained. The sera were separated and preserved at -20 °C in HIPH lab

All samples were undergone third generation ELISA test,(WKEA, China).

Principle of the assay:

Anti-HCV employs solid phase, indirect ELISA method for detection of antibodies to HCV in two-step incubation procedure. Polystyrene microwell strips are pre-coated with recombinant, highly immunoreactive antigens corresponding to the core and the non-structural regions of HCV (NS3, NS4, NS5). During the first incubation step, anti-HCV specific antibodies, if present, will be bound to the solid phase pre-coated HCV antigens. The wells were washed to remove unbound serum proteins, and rabbit anti-human IgG antibodies (anti-IgG) conjugated to the enzyme horseradish peroxidase (HRP-Conjugate) are added. During the second incubation step, these HRP-conjugated antibodies will be bound to any antigen-antibody(IgG) complexes previously formed and the unbound HRP-conjugate is then removed by washing.

Chromogen solutions containing tetramethylbenzidine (TMB) and urea peroxide are added to the wells and in presence of the antigen-antibody-anti-IgG (HRP) immunocomplex, the colorless chromogens are hydrolyzed by the bound HRP conjugate to a blue-colored product. The blue color turns yellow after stopping the reaction with sulfuric acid. The amount of color intensity can be measured and it is proportional to the amount of antibody in the sample respectively. Wells containing samples negative for anti-HCV remain colorless.

Calculation of the cut-off value(C.O) =*Nc + 0.12

*Nc = the mean absorbance value for three negative controls.

All study participants were informed about their results. Only those who were positive for HCVAb were invited to provide blood samples for the following tests:

1. PCR test (Real-time cobas amplipred cobas Taqman)
2. ELISA for hepatitis B virus surface antigen (HBs-Ag) test.(Dialab, Austria)

Principles of HBs-Ag test:

HBsAg ELISA uses polystyrene microwell strips pre-coated with monoclonal antibodies specific to HBsAg. Patient's serum or plasma sample is added to the microwelltogether with a second antibody conjugatedwith horseradish peroxidase (HRP) and directed against a different epitope of HBsAg. During incubation, the specific immunocomplex formed in case of presence of HBsAg in the sample, is captured on the solid phase. After washing to remove sample serum proteins and unbound HRP-conjugate, Chromogen solutions containing tetramethylbenzidine (TMB)and urea peroxide are added to the wells . In presence of the antibody-antigen-antibody(HRP) "sandwich" immunocomplex , the colorless Chromogens are hydrolysedby the bound HRP-conjugate to a blue colored product. The blue color turns yellow after stopping the reaction with sulfuric acid. The amount of color can be measured and is proportional to stopping the reaction with sulfuric acid. The amount of color can be measured and is proportional to the amount of antigen in the sample. Wells containing samples negative for HBsAg remain colorless.

3. ELISA for Hepatitis B virus anicore antibody (HBc-Ab) test.(DIALAB Austria)

Principles of HBc-Ab test:

This anti-HBc ELISA KIT is based on solid phase, one step incubation competitive principle ELISA.Anti-HBc if present in the sample competes with monoclonal anti-HBc conjugated to horseradish peroxidase (HRP) for a fixed amount of purified HBcAg pre-coated in the wells. When no anti-HBc presents in the sample, the HRP labeled

Anti-HBc will bound with the antigens inside the wells and any unbound HRP-conjugate is removed during washing. Chromogen B and A solutions are added into the wells and during incubation, the colorless Chromogens are hydrolyzed by the bound HRP-Conjugate to a blue colored product. The blue color turns yellow after stopping the reaction with sulfuric acid. No or low color developing suggests the presence of antibodies to HBcAg in sample.

Statistical analysis:

The collected data was revised, coded, entered to personal computer and finally analyzed using SPSS (statistics package for social science) Version 15. Data were fed to the computer using the Predictive Analytics Software *(PASW Statistics 18)*.

Qualitative data were described using number and percent. Association between categorical variables was tested using *Chi-square test*. When more than 20% of the cells have expected count less than 5, correction for chi-square was conducted using *Firsher's Exact test* or *Monte Carlo correction*.

Quantitative data were described using median, minimum and maximum as well as mean and standard deviation.

The distributions of quantitative variables were tested for normality using *Kolmogorov-Smirnov test, Shapiro-Wilk test. D'Agstino test* was used if there was a conflict between the two previous tests. If it reveals normal data distribution, parametric tests was applied. If the data were abnormally distributed, non-parametric tests were used.

For normally distributed data, comparison between two independent population were done using *independent t-test.*

Significance test results are quoted as two-tailed probabilities. Significance of the obtained results was judged at the 5% level.

RESULTS

RESULTS

During the 4 months recruitment period, 360 women consented to participate in the present study. Of them only 22 found to be positive for HCV antibodies on screening using third generation ELISA technique indicating a sample prevalence of 6.1% (95% confidence interval = 3.87-9.11) (Fig.1).

The prevalence in different villages is shown in table 1. About 77.3% (17/22) of the HCV Ab positive women were found in 4 villages out of the total 9 villages ; Abo-elyosr, Adam, Malek and Belal. The highest prevalence was found in Abo-elyosr and Adam (22.7%) in each. The least prevalence was found in Solyman village with no cases there (p = 0.260). (fig.2).

Table (1): Prevalence of HCVAbs in different villages

Village name	Total	HCV Abs				^{MC}p
		-ve (n = 388)		+ve (n = 22)		
		No.	%	No.	%	
Belal	32	29	90.6	3	9.4	
Solyman	13	13	100.0	0	0.0	
Abo-elyosr	33	28	84.8	5	15.2	
Abd elwahab	53	51	96.2	2	3.8	
Abd elrakeeb	12	11	91.7	1	8.3	0.260
Malek	62	58	93.5	4	6.5	
Elishaa	50	49	98.0	1	2.0	
Yousef	47	46	97.9	1	2.1	
Adam	58	53	91.4	5	8.6	

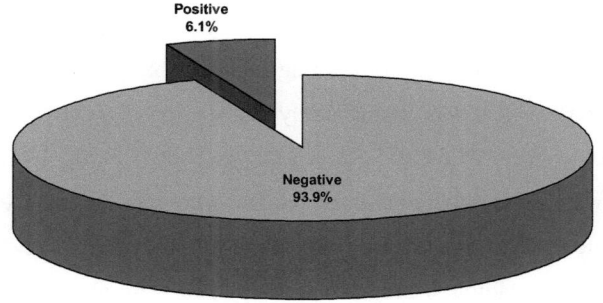

Figure (1): Distribution of the pregnant women according to HCVAbs

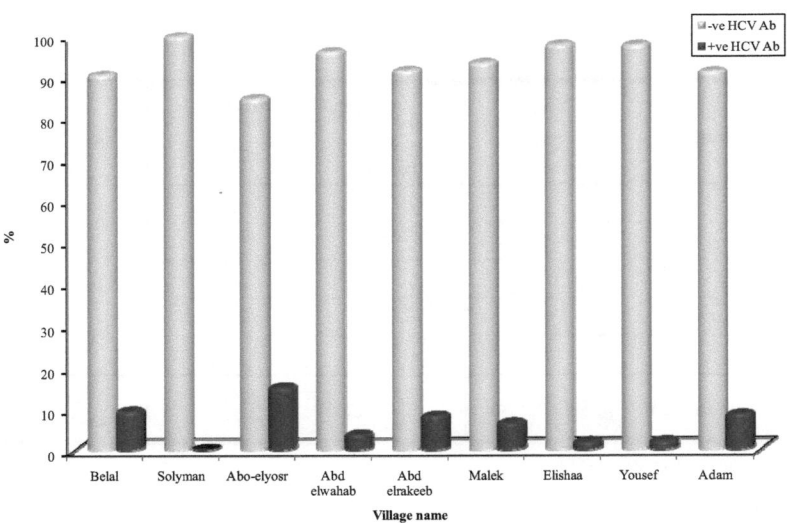

Figure (2): Prevalence of HCV Ab in different villages

18

Participants ranged in age from 16 to 45 years old, ($\bar{x}$ = 25.87 ± 5.81 years).As shown in Figure 2 the mean age for HCVAb positive women was (28.59 ± 6.63) which was significantly higher (p= 0.023) than HCVAb negative women ($\bar{x}$= 25.69 ± 5.72 years). As shown in fig.4; the highest prevalence was found among pregnant women who was above 35 years old (13.2%) while the least prevalence was found in those who was between 20-25 years (2.3 %). Although pregnant women who were above 30 years old constitute about one fourth of the studied population, they contributed to more than half of those proved to be HCVAb positive.(fig.3)

Table (2): Prevalence of the pregnant women in different age groups.

Age group	Total	HCV Ab Positive		Test of sig.
	No. (n=360)	No. (n=22)	%	
<20	39	3	7.7	
20-	128	3	2.3	
25-	100	4	4.0	$^{MC}p = 0.014^{*}$
30-	55	7	12.7	
35+	38	5	13.2	
Mean ± SD	25.87 ± 5.82	28.59 ± 6.63		$t = 2.281^{*}$ $p = 0.023$

^{MC}p: p value for Monte Carlo test
t: Student t-test
*: Statistically significant at p ≤0.05

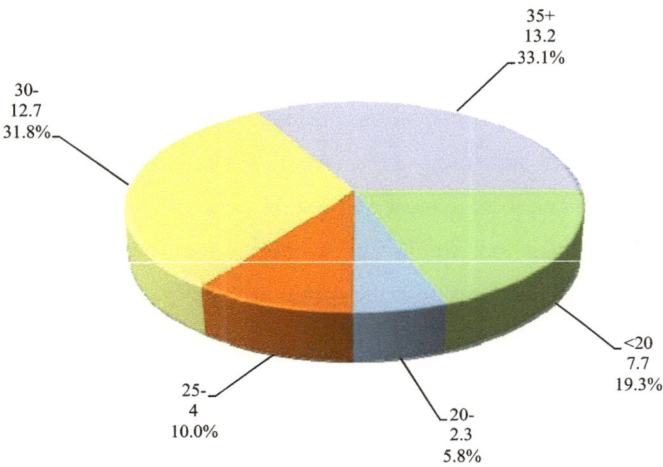

Figure (3): Distribution of the pregnant women according to the prevalence of HCV Abs among each age group.

About one third of the participant women were illiterate and another one third had secondary school education with no significant difference between seronegative and seropositive women. About 96.4% of the surveyed women were housewives and only 3.6% were working. Twenty one of the seropositive women were housewives and only one of them was a health care worker. There was no significant difference between seropositive and seronegative women regarding to the nature of work (p value = 0.567).

Table (3): Distribution of the pregnant women according to sociodemographic characteristics

Sociodemographic characteristics	Total	HCV Ab				Test of significance	
		Negative (n=338)		Positive (n=22)			
		No.	%	No.	%		
Education							
Illiterate	122	116	95.1	6	4.9		
Read and Write	5	4	80.0	1	20.0		
Primary	41	37	90.2	4	9.8		
Middle	60	57	95.0	3	5.0	MCP=	0.516
Secondary	121	113	93.4	8	6.6		
University	11	11	100.0	0	0.0		
Work							
Housewife	347	326	93.9	21	6.1		
Health care worker	4	3	75.0	1	25.0		
Employee	4	4	100.0	0	0.0	MCP=	0.567
Clinical Laboratory worker	1	1	100.0	0	0.0		
Others	4	4	100.0	0	0.0		

Table 4 illustrates that none of the potential HCV risk behaviour had a relation with the presence of HCVAb in the study participants. Moreover there was no correlation between the number of risk factors (positive for no risk factors, one risk factor, two risk factors) and the likelihood of being HCV positive (p > 0.05).

Table (4): Distribution of the pregnant women according to the risk factors for HCV

| Risk factors for HCV | Total | HCV Ab | | | | Test of significance |
| | | Negative (n=338) | | Positive (n=22) | | |
		No.	%	No.	%	
Undergone surgery						
No	216	204	94.4	12	5.6	X^2= 0.29
Yes	144	134	93.1	10	6.9	p= 0.590
Had blood or blood product transfusion						
No	345	326	94.5	19	5.5	FETp= 0.056
Yes (After 1992)	15	12	80.0	3	20.0	
Undergone dental manipulation						
No	158	148	93.7	10	6.3	X^2= 0.02
Yes	202	190	94.1	12	5.9	p= 0.879
Suffering from accident or injury						
No	352	331	94.0	21	6.0	FETp= 0.399
Yes	8	7	87.5	1	12.5	
Ear Piercing						
No	14	8	57.1	6	42.9	FETp= 0.000
Yes	346	330	95.4	16	4.6	
Sharing razors, tooth brush, or any item that could carry infected blood						
No	159	148	93.1	11	6.9	X^2= 0.32
Yes	201	190	94.5	11	5.5	p= 0.570
Female Circumcision						
No	32	30	93.8	2	6.3	FETp= 0.999
Yes	328	308	93.9	20	6.1	
Had hijama						
No	344	323	93.9	21	6.1	FETp= 0.999
Yes	16	15	93.8	1	6.3	
Injected intravenous medications						
No	105	100	95.2	5	4.8	X^2= 0.47
Yes	255	238	93.3	17	6.7	p= 0.493

None of the items of previous gestational history was significantly associated with HCVAb presence (Table 5). These items included (number of the previous pregnancies, history of bleeding during pregnancy , type of previous labour and medical history related to pregnancy).

Table (5): Distribution of the pregnant women according to their past antenatal history

Previous Gestational History	Total	HCV Ab				Test of significance	
		Negative (n=338)		Positive (n=22)			
		No.	%	No.	%		
Number of previous pregnancies							
Less than 3	167	233	94.3	14	5.7		
3 or more	113	105	92.9	8	7.1		
Mean ± SD (Median)	*1.97 ± 1.73 (2.0)*	*1.94 ± 1.69 (2.0)*		*2.45 ± 2.2 (2.0)*		t= p=	1.07 0.293
History of bleeding during pregnancy							
No	320	299	93.4	21	6.6	FETp=	0.490
Yes	40	39	97.5	1	2.5		
Type of previous labour							
Normal vaginal delivery	232	217	93.5	15	6.5	p=	0.881
Caesarean	59	55	93.2	4	6.8	p=	0.949
DC	22	21	95.5	1	4.5	p=	0.891
Abortion without DC	44	43	97.7	1	2.3	p=	0.422
Medical history related to pregnancy							
No	316	296	93.7	20	6.3		
Hypertension	9	8	88.9	1	11.1		
DM	2	2	100.0	0	0.0	MCP=	0.560
Bleeding	32	31	96.9	1	3.1		
Hypertension + Bleeding	1	1	100.0	0	0.0		

The sociodemographic data of the husbands are shown in Table 6. Their ages ranged from 18 to 65 years old ($\bar{x} = 31.83 \pm 7.42$ years), most of them (52.8%) were between 25-35 years old. It is evident in Figure 4 that the mean age for HCVAb positive women husbands was significantly higher (p = 0.013) than that of HCVAb negative husbands ($\bar{x} = 37.09 \pm 9.53$ versus 31.48 ± 7.14 respectively).

More than one quarter (27.2%) of the studied husbands were illiterate, those who reached secondary education constituted 37.5%. Only 8.6% had a university degree. The educational levels were distributed normally between both groups (Fig.5) except for those who can only read and write (50% in each group; p = 0.007). Meanwhile, the type of work of the husbands did not differ significantly between both groups.

Table (6):   Distribution   of   the   studied   sample   according   to Sociodemographic characteristics of the husband

Sociodemographic characteristics of the husband	Total	HCV Ab				Test of significance	
		Negative (n=338)		Positive (n=22)			
		No.	%	No.	%		
ge in years							
<25	53	51	96.2	2	3.8		
25-	190	184	96.8	6	3.2	$X^2=$	17.231[*]
35-	84	77	91.7	7	8.3	p=	0.001
45+	33	26	78.8	7	21.2		
Mean ± SD	31.83 ± 7.42	31.48 ± 7.14		37.09 ± 9.53		t=	2.71
(Median)	(30.0)	(30.0)		(35.0)		p=	0.013
Education							
Illiterate	98	91	92.9	7	7.1		
Read and Write	8	4	50.0	4	50.0		
Primary	41	39	95.1	2	4.9	MCP=	0.007
Middle	47	45	95.7	2	4.3		
Secondary	135	129	95.6	6	4.4		
University	31	30	96.8	1	3.2		
Work							
Farmer	229	215	93.9	14	6.1		
Clerk	39	37	94.9	2	5.1		
Manual	33	31	93.9	2	6.1	MCP=	0.898
Professional	14	14	100.0	0	0.0		
Others	45	41	91.1	4	8.9		

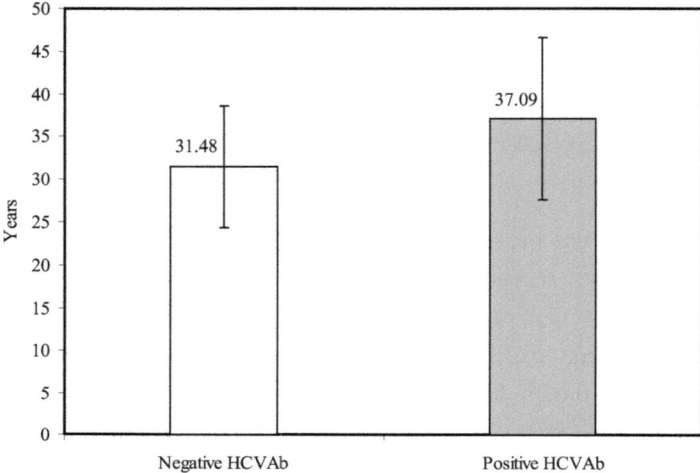

Figure (4): Distribution of the studied pregnant women to the mean age of the husband and HCV Abs

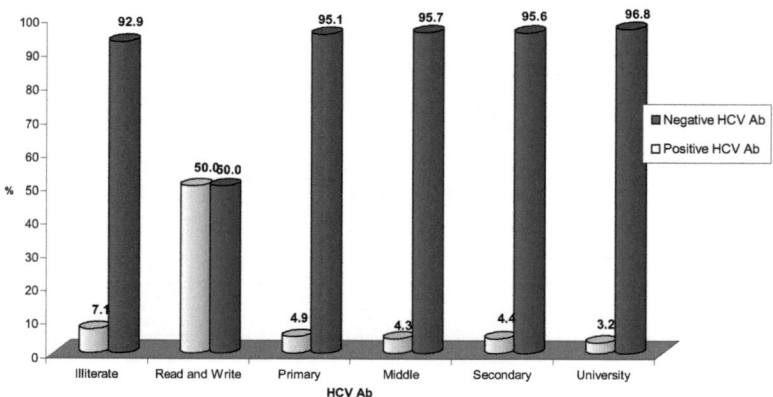

Figure (5): Distribution of the pregnant women according to education of the husband and HCV Abs

Table 7 demonstrates the distribution of the studied sample according to risk factors of HCV in the husbands. The percentage of HCV negative women whose husbands did not have any dental manouver was higher than those who gave such a history (96.6% versus 91.9%) respectively. Although seventeen (8.1%) of the women whose husbands have undergone dental manipulation were HCVAb positive compared to only five (3.4%) of those who denied any dental manouvers, it did not reach a statistically significant level (p= 0.067). Husbands who reported tattoing , intravenous medications, surgical operation were not significantly associated with HCVAb status of their wives.

History of chronic liver disease in the husbands was significantly associated with HCVAbs presence in the wives. As shown in Figure 7 about one third of those who reported chronic liver disease were among the husbands of HCVAb positive group(p= 0.018).

Table (7): Distribution of the studied sample according to risk factors of HCV in the husband

Risk factors for HCV	Total	HCV Ab				Test of significance	
		Negative (n=338)		Positive (n=22)			
		No.	%	No.	%		
Dental manouvers							
No	149	144	96.6	5	3.4	X^2=	3.36
Yes	211	194	91.9	17	8.1	p=	0.067
Tattoing							
No	343	321	93.6	22	6.4	FETp=	0.612
Yes	17	17	100.0	0	0.0		
Intravenous drug use							
No	345	324	93.9	21	6.1	FETp=	0.999
Yes	15	14	93.3	1	6.7		
Surgical operation							
No	269	253	94.1	16	5.9	X^2=	0.05
Yes	91	85	93.4	6	6.6	p=	0.824
Chronic liver disease							
No	350	331	94.6	19	5.4	FETp=	0.018
Yes	10	7	70.0	3	30.0		

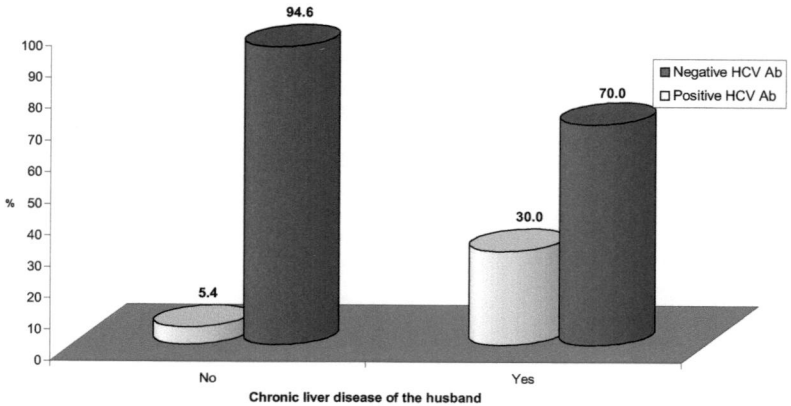

Figure (6): Distribution of the pregnant women according to prescence of chronic liver disease in the husband and HCV Abs

27

Regarding the presence of HCV viraemia as detected by real time PCR, only 20 out of the 22 HCV positive pregnant women consented to have this test. Less than half of them (9/20; 45%) had viraemia. The viraemia ranged from 1.3×10^{2} to 2.7×10^{6} with a mean $\pm$ SD of $4.7 \times 10^{5} \pm (8.78 \times 10^{5})$.

Only one (4.5%) had a detectable HBsAg and 4 (18.2%) had evidence of exposure to HBV as indicated by detection of (anti-HBc).

Table 8 refers to the relationship between PCR results and the different parameters of the pregnant women. Seven women (77.8%) of the PCR positive women were above 30 years and none was detected among those between 20-30 years old. The difference in age between both groups did not reach a statistically significant level (p = 0.062).

Women who were PCR positive and undergone dental manipulation were about 66.7% of all positive cases which also had not a significant difference between PCR positive and PCR negative women (p = 0.177).

Positive PCR women who shared razors, tooth brushes or any item that could carry infected blood was also 66.7% (6 women) of the total positive PCR women with no significant difference between PCR positive and PCR negative women (p = 0.406).

66.6% of the positive PCR women were pregnant previously from 2 to 4 times before (p = 0.338).

Table (8): Relationship between PCR results and different parameters of pregnant women

	PCR				Test of sig.
	-ve (n = 11)		+ve (n = 9)		
	No.	%	No.	%	
Age					
<20	1	9.1	2	22.2	
20-	3	27.3	0	0.0	MCp =
25-	3	27.3	0	0.0	0.062
30-	1	9.1	5	55.6	
35+	3	27.3	2	22.2	
Mean ± SD	27.82 ± 6.95		29.78 ± 6.91		p = 0.543
Education					
Illiterate	2	18.2	4	44.4	
Read and write	1	9.1	0	0.0	MCp =
Primary	2	18.2	1	11.1	0.576
Middle	2	18.2	0	0.0	
Secondary	4	36.4	4	44.4	
Undergone surgery					
No	6	45.5	6	44.4	MCp =
Minor	0	0.0	1	11.1	0.818
Mojor	5	45.5	4	44.4	
Had blood or blood production transfusion					
No	10	90.9	7	77.8	FEp =
Yes (After 1992)	1	9.1	2	22.0	0.566
Undergone dental manipulation					
No	7	63.6	3	33.3	MCp =
Infrequent	1	9.1	0	0.0	0.177
Frequent	3	27.3	6	66.7	
Sharing razors, tooth brush, or any item that could carry infected blood					
No	6	54.5	3	33.3	FEp =
Yes	5	45.5	6	66.7	0.406
Number of pervious pregnancies	2.18 ± 1.94		3.0 ± 2.69		p = 0.440
0	1	9.1	2	22.2	
1	4	36.4	0	0.0	
2	3	27.3	2	22.2	
3	1	9.1	2	22.2	MCp =
4	1	9.1	2	22.2	0.338
7	1	9.1	0	0.0	
9	0	0.0	1	11.0	
History of bleeding during pregnancy					
No	10	90.9	9	100.0	FEp =
Yes	1	9.1	0	0.0	1.000
Medical history related to pregnancy					
None	10	90.9	8	88.9	MCp =
HTN	0	0.0	1	11.1	0.713
Bleeding	1	9.1	0	0.0	

29

No significant results were detected between prevalence of viraemia and the educational, potential risk factors of hepatitis or obstetric history of the pregnant women.

Table 9 illustrates the relationship between PCR results of the pregnant women and the different parameters of their husbands. According to the age of the husbands of PCR positive women, about 77.7% of them were above 35 years but there was no significant difference between ages of husbands of PCR positive and PCR negative women (p = 0.106).

Most of the husbands (66.6%) of PCR positive women had educational level between middle, secondary or university degree with no statistically significant difference with husbands of PCR negative women (p = 0.465).

Table (9): Relationship between PCR and different parameters of husbands

	PCR				Test of sig.
	-ve (n = 11)		+ve (n = 9)		
	No.	%	No.	%	
Age					
<25	0	0.0	2	22.2	
25-	4	36.4	0	0.0	MCp = 0.106
35	4	36.4	3	33.3	
45+	3	27.3	4	44.4	
Mean ± SD	37.18 ± 10.07		37.89 ± 9.92		p = 0.879
Education					
Illiterate	4	36.4	2	22.2	
Read and write	3	27.3	1	11.1	
Primary	1	9.1	0	0.0	MCp = 0.465
Middle	0	0.0	2	22.2	
Secondary	3	27.3	3	33.3	
University	0	0.0	1	11.1	
Work					
Farmer	5	45.5	7	77.8	
Clerk	2	18.2	0	0.0	MCp = 0.617
Manual	1	9.1	1	11.1	
tOthers	3	27.3	1	11.1	
Dental manouvers of husband					
No	3	27.2	2	22.2	FEp = 1.000
Yes	8	72.7	7	77.8	
Surgical operation of husband					
No	9	81.8	6	66.7	FEp = 0.617
Yes	2	18.2	3	33.3	
Chronic liver disease of husband					
No	9	81.8	8	88.9	FEp = 1.000
Yes	2	18.2	1	11.1	
HBS Ag					
Negative	11	100.0	8	88.9	FEp = 0.450
Positive	0	0.0	1	11.1	
HBV anticore					
Not done	0	0.0	1	11.1	
Negative	9	81.8	6	66.7	MCp = 0.773
Positive	2	18.2	2	22.2	
Type of previous labour					
Normal	7	70.0	6	85.7	
Cesarean	2	20.0	2	28.6	
DC	1	10.0	0	0.0	-
Abortion without DC	1	10.0	0	0.0	

DISCUSSION

DISCUSSION

In this study 6.1% of the participants were positive for HCV-Ab, this prevalence rate is lower than that reported before in other similar studies as in 2006 Abdel-Hamid et al reported a prevalence of 15.8% (408 out of 2587 women) among the pregnant women in the rural Delta region[25]. A study at 2010 in Assiut by Zahran et al reported a prevalence of 11.7% among 500 *pregnant* women[31]. In Benha Khaled AbdulQawi et al in 2012 found that out of 1224 pregnant women 105 were seropositive for HCV antibody 8.6% (95% confidence interval, 7.05-10.17)[32].

Although the prevalence of HCV in Egypt appears to have decreased, our prevalence of 6.1% is still higher than in other countries such as the USA (3.2%), Taiwan (1.5%), Zaire (6%)[32].

In Egypt demographic health survey (DHS) 2008 the prevalence among women was 12.2 % out of that aged 15-59 years old[33].

In Saudi Arabia Ghazi in 2007 reported a prevalence which was close to our prevalence as out of 2160 pregnant women, 114 were seropositive at their first antenatal visit, making the seroprevalence rate 6.66 % while the prevalence in genral population is ranging from 1.0% to 6.9% (Saudi show lower prevalence (1.0-5.0%) than non-Saudis (1.7-6.9%)[34].

A similar research had been conducted in Pakistan 2009 Shaikh et al found that the prevalence was 3.44%[35]; while it was 4.95% ± 0.53% in the general population[36]. But our results is much higher than some other developing countries like India as in 2007 Ashok Kumar et al reported that the prevalence was 1.03% (Eighty four) out of 8130 pregnant women were positive for anti-HCV antibodies compared to 1-1.9 among general population[37]. In Nigeria Clement et al reported that anti-HCV Ab was only detected in 2 out of the 506 (0.4%) pregnant women [38]. compared to 4.7% among general population[39].

In the developed countries the prevalence is so much lower than that of Egypt, In Canada 2010 Collen et al found that the prevalence was 0.5 % among pregnant women[40]. In Central Brazil out of 28,561 pregnant women were screened by Costa et al for HCV-Ab the Prevalence of HCV infection was 0.15% (95% CI 0.11%–0.20%)[41].

Our study showed that the most important risk factors for HCV infection among pregnant women were older age of the pregnant woman, older age of the husband and chronic liver disease of the husband.

This study included women ranging in age from 16 to 45 years, with a mean age (25.87 ± 5.81 years). Abdukqawi et al study was carried out among 1224 pregnant women (mean age 25.3± 5.1 years; range, 16-45 years) they found an association between HCV infection and older age [32]. Our results are also in agreement with Costa et al, who indicated that HCV is associated with older age as out of 28,576 pregnant women only 40 women were HCV seropositive and their ages range between12-40 years old ((mean = 23.9; sd = 5.6) , the majority of seropositve women was among those who was 20-40 years old (90%)[41]. In contrast to our results Zahran et al reported that there were no significant differences in mean age of the pregnant women [31].

Higher rate of infection among older age group can be explained by cohort phenomenon and the cumulative effect of exposure to HCV due to the long period of viral exposure over one's lifetime, as well as exposure to other potential HCV risk factors.

Surprisingly, none of the potential HCV risk behavior of the pregnant women had a relation with the presence of HCV-Ab in the study participants. But we found a significant association between seropositivity and husband age and being a chronic liver disease patient which rise our caution regarding the route of transmission.

According to this study blood transfusion had a respectable association with HCV infection but it did not reach a significant value as pregnant women who previously received blood transfusion and have HCV-Ab were 0.83 % of all screened women, while those who received blood but have not HCV-Ab were 3.33 % of all screened women. These findings closely coincide with that of Ashok Kumar et al (4.8 % of HCV-Ab had blood transfusion versus 3.1 % among HCV-Ab negative) [37]. In contrast Kamal M et al reported a history of blood transfusion in 6.6% of HCV-Ab positive versus 2.2% in those who were negative [31]. AbdulQawi Kh et al also found blood transfusion as a risk factor for infection (15% of HCV-Ab positive women had transfusion versus 3.9 % among HCV-Ab negative women) [32].

The cause that made the blood transfusion is not an effective risk factor in the present study may be due to the mandatory testing of blood donors and blood products.

According to ages of husbands of the participating pregnant women the mean age for HCV-Ab positive women husbands was significantly higher (p = 0.013) than that of HCV-Ab negative husbands ($\bar{x}$ = 37.09 ± 9.53 versus 31.48 ±7.14 respectively).

Dental maneuvers of the husband had a respectable association with HCV infection but it did not reach a significant value.

SUMMARY

SUMMARY

Hepatitis C virus infection is considered a highly spread infection. It is estimated that 130-170 million people is infected with HCV infection world-wide. It is considered the main cause of chronic hepatitis, fibrosis and hepatocellular carcinoma.

In Egypt HCV infection is considered a major health burden as it is the highest rate in the world as it is estimated 14.7% from the general population.

The ideal treatment for HCV infection is a combination between interferon and ribavirin.

Pregnancy may be an important time to screen for HCV infection. Many women will already have reached their peak likelihood of becoming infected by the time they become pregnant, making the yield of testing near its maximum. Further, testing for HCV during pregnancy may help to identify infected newborns, allowing for appropriate follow-up.

The research was carried out in randomly selected 9 villages affiliated to Al-nobareya town in Albehiera governorate, 360 pregnant women shared in the research in 1 18 weeks period after a consent from every woman.

All pregnant women who accepted to participate were inserted whatever their gestation period , and we excluded that who has known HCV infection or chronic liver disease.

A pre designed questionnaire was filled. It contained data regarding socio-demographic and contact data (name, age, occupation, education, address, telephone number) and data regarding possible risk factors (history of operation, dental procedure, blood transfusion, tattooing, circumcision, intravenous drugs, invasive procedures, HCV +ve husband, family history, etc). A five ml blood sample was withdrawn using the universal sterile precautions. Each visit 20-30 samples were obtained. The sera were separated and preserved at -20 °C in HIPH lab. All samples were undergone third generation ELISA test.

Only those who were positive for HCV-Ab were invited to provide blood samples for PCR test and ELISA for hepatitis B virus surface antigen (HBs-Ag) test.

Out of 360 women consented to participate in the present study only 22 found to be positive for HCV antibodies on indicating a sample prevalence of 6.1%.

The research was cleared that there is a significant statistical relationship between the presence of HCV-Ab in the serum and the following risk factors (increase age of the pregnant woman, increase age of the husband and presence of chronic liver disease in the husband). But the research failed to provide is a significant statistical relationship between the presence of HCV-Ab in the serum and the other risk factors.

CONCLUSION

CONCLUSION

The prevalence of HCV infection in pregnant women in Egypt is lower than previously reported. The detected risk factors are age of the pregnant women, age of their husbands and chronic liver disease of the husbands. None of the other known risk factors was found to be significantly associated with the HCV infection.

RECOMMENDATION

RECOMMENDATION

We recommend doing further research containing a larger sample to detect the other most important risk factors for HCV-Ab seropositive.

REFERENCES

REFERENCES

1. Houghton M. The long and winding road leading to the identification of the hepatitis C virus.Hepatol.2009; 51 (5): 939–48.

2. Pondé RA. Hidden hazards of HCV transmission. Immunol Med Mic. 2011;200 (1): 7–11.

3. WHO. Cancer.[Cited 2012 February] Fact sheet number 297.

4. Wilkins T, Malcolm JK, Raina D, Schade RR. Hepatitis C: diagnosis and treatment. Am Fam Phys.2010; 81 (11): 1351–7.

5. Holmberg SC, Brunette GW, Kozarsky PE, Magill AJ. Health information for international travel. Oxford University Press. 2012;12: 231.

6. WHO. Hepatitis C. [Cited July 2012]. Fact sheet number 164.

7. Miller FD, Abu-Raddad. The Hepatitis C Virus Epidemic in Egypt. Proc Natl. 2010; 10:1073.

8. Alter MJ. Sporadic non-A, non-B hepatitis: frequency and epidemiology in an urban United States population. J Infect Dis. 1982; 145:886-893.

9. Stramer SL. Detection of HIV-1 and HCV infections among antibody-negative blood donors by nucleic acid-amplification testing. N Engl Med 2004; 351:760-768.

10. Eijaz GH, Muhammad AY. NAT for HCV Screening in Blood Banking. Pak Armed Forces Med J. 2006;56(4):438-40.

11. Garfein RS. Viral infections in short-term injection drug users: the prevalence of the hepatitis C, hepatitis B, human immunodeficiency, and human T-lymphotropic viruses. Am J Public Health 1996; 86:655-671.

12. CDC. Recommendations for prevention and control of hepatitis C virus (HCV) infection and HCV-related chronic disease. *MMWR*1998;47(19):1-39.

13. Patrick DM. Public health and hepatitis C. Can J Public 2000;91(1): 18-23.

14. Hahn JA. Hepatitis C virus infection and needle exchange use among young injection drug users in San Francisco.Hepatol. 2001;34: 180-7.

15. Conry CC. Routes of infection, viremia, and liver disease in blood donors found to have hepatitis C virus infection. N Engl J Med 1996; 334:1691-6.

16. Gross JB. Hepatitis C: A sexually transmitted disease?. Am J Gastroenterol. 2001; 96:3051-3.

17. Vandelli C, Renzo F, Romano L, Tisminetzky S, Palma M. Lack of evidence of sexual transmission of hepatitis C among monogamous couples: results of a 10-year prospective follow-up study. Am J Gastroenterol.2004; 99:855-9.

18. Terrault NA.Sexual activity as a risk factor for epatitis.Hepatol.2002; 36:99-105.

19. Indolfi G, Bartolini E, Casavola D. Chronic hepatitis C virus infection in children and adolescents. Dove Press .2010; 2010: 115 –28.

20. Mohamed MK, Abdel-Hamid, Mikhail NN. Intrafamilial transmission of hepatitis C in Egypt. Hepatol.2005;42(3)683-7.

21. Ackerman Z, Ackerman E, Paltiel O. Intrafamilial transmission of hepatitis C virus: a systematic review .Viral Hepatol.2000;7:93-103.

22. Carli DG, Puro V, Ippolito G. Risk of hepatitis C virus transmission following percutaneous exposure in healthcare workers. Infection 2003; 31(2):22-7.

23. Sulkowski MS, Ray SC, Thomas DL. Needlestick transmission of hepatitis C.JAMA 2002;287:2406-13.

24. Flamm SL, Parker RA, Chopra S. Risk factors associated with chronic hepatitis C virus infection: limited frequency of an unidentified source of transmission. Am J Gastroenterol. 1998; 93:597-600.

25. Stoszek SK, Abdel-Hamid M, Narooz SH. Prevalence of and risk factors for hepatitis C in rural pregnant Egyptian women. R Soc Trop Med Hyg. 2006; 100(2): 102-7.

26. Newell ML, Pembrey L. Mother-to-child transmission of hepatitis C virus infection. Drugs Today 2002, 38(5): 321-3.

27. Barakat SH, EL-Bashir NB. Hepatitis C virus infection among healthy Egyptian children: prevalence and risk factors. Viral Hepatol. 2011;18(11):779-84.

28. Rosenthal P. Is our approach to treating chronic hepatitis C all wrong? J. Pediatr Gastroenterol Nutr. 2009; 31:100.

29. Jacobson KR, Murray K, Zellos A, Schwarz KB. An analysis of published trials of interferon monotherapy in children with chronic hepatitis C. Pediatr Gastroenterol Nutr. 2002; 34:52-8.

30. CDC. National Prevention Strategy,2001. Houghton M. The long and winding road leading to the identification of the hepatitis C virus. J Hepatol 2009; 51(5): 939–948.

31. Zahran KM, Badary MS, Agban MN, Abdel Aziz NH.. Pattern of hepatitis virus infection among pregnant women and their newborns at the Women's Health Center of Assiut University, Upper Egypt. Int J Gynaecol Obstet 2010; 11: 171-174.

32. AbdulQawi Kh, Youssef A, Metwally A, RagihI, Abduelhamid M, Shaheen A. Prospective study of prevalence and risk factors of Hepatitis C in pregnant Egyptian women and its transmission to their infants. Croat Med J 2010; 51: 219-228.

33. Egypt DHS 2008. 251-258.

34. Ghazi O. Hepatitis C virus in pregnancy in Kingdom of Saudi Arabia. J Sci Med Eng 2007; 19:137-144.

35. Shaikh F, Naqvi SQ, Jilani K, Memon RA. Prevalence and risk factors of Hepatitis C virus during pregnancy. Gomal J Med 2009; 7: 86-87.

36. Yasir W, Talha Sh, Sher Z, Ishtiaq Q. Hepatitis C virus in Pakistan: A systematic review of prevalence, genotypes and risk factors. World J Gastroenterol2009;7:5647-5653.

37. Kumar A, Sharma KA, Gupta RK, Kar P, Chakravarti A. Prevalence and risk factors for hepatitis C virus among pregnant women. Indian J M ed Res 2007; 126: 211-215.

38. Clement MI, Andy EI, Eni LO, Jewell PA. Prevalence, sociodemographic characterestics and risk factors for Hepatitis C infection among pregnant women in Calabar, Municipality, Nigeria. Hepat Mon 2010; 10: 116–120.

39. Olive O, Sylvester N, Abraham M, Olufunmilayo A. Risk Factors for Hepatitis C Virus Transmission Obscure in Nigerian Patients. Gastroenterol Res Pract 2011;10:1155-1159.

40. Collen D, Cathrien C, Mark H. The effectiveness of screening of Hepatitis C virus in pregnancy. JOGC 2010;32(11):1035-1041.

41. Costa ZB , Machado GC, Avelino MM, et al. pregnant Prevalence and risk factors for Hepatitis C and HIV-1 infections among women in Central Brazil. BMC infect Dis.2009;9:116.

الملخص العربى

الملخص العربى

تعتبر نسبة الإصابة بفيروس الالتهاب الكبدى (سي) مرتفعة للغاية وتقدر عدد الاصابات حوالى من 130 الى ١٧٠ مليون نسمة في جميع أنحاء العالم ويعد هو السبب الرئيسى للإصابة بمرض الالتهاب الكبدى الرمز من وتليف الكبد والأورام الكبدية.

فـي مصـر يشـكل انتشـار عـدوى التهـاب الكبـد الوبائى المزمن (سـي) مشكلة صحـية كبـرى حيـث أنها هـي الاعلـى فـي معدلات الإصابـة بهـذا المرض في العالم حيـث تبلـغ النسبة العامة لمعدل انتشار الإصابة بالفيروس حوالي 14.7 ٪

يعتبر العلاج الأمثل لمرضى الالتهاب الكبدى الوبائى المزمن (سي) هو الجمع بين عقارى الانتيرفيرون طويل المفعول والريبافيرين.

وتعتبر فترة الحمل من أكثر الفترات المهم فيها التحري عن وجود الالتهاب الكبدي الفيروسي سي حيث أن الكثير من السيدات يصلن إلى ذروة فرص ظهور الفيروس في فترة الحمل كما أن التعرف على وجود اللالتهاب الكبدي في تلك الفترة يساعد كثيرا في بدء العلاج في وقت مناسب وكذلك توخي الحذر من أجل عدم نقل العدوى للمولود الجديد.

أجريت الدراسة في الوحدات الصحية في تسعة من القرى التابعة لمدينة النوبارية بمحافظة البحيرة على 360 سيدة حامل في خلال 18 أسبوع وذلك بعد الحصول على الموافقة من كل مريضة.

تم إدراج جميع السيدات الحوامل اللاتي وافقن على الاشتراك في الدراسة بغض النظر عن عدد أشهر الحمل وتم استبعاد من تعرف مسبقا بوجود الفيروس لديها أو أي مرض كبدي مزمن.

تم ملئ استبيان معد مسبقا بواسطة الباحث يحتوي على المعلومات الشخصية التالية (الاسم- العمر- الوظيفة – مستوى التعليم- العنوان- رقم الهاتف).

كذلك تم السؤال عن العوامل التنبؤية المتمثلة في (عمليات جراحية سابقة- إجراءات طبية للأسنان- نقل دم- وشم- ختان- أدوية وريدية- زوج حامل للفيروس- تاريخ مرضي للفيروس داخل العائلة).

تم جمع عينات الدم بواسطة سرنجات معقمة بمعدل 30-20 حالة في الزيارة الواحدة وتم فصل السيرام وتجميده عند درجة حرارة 20 منوية تحت الصفر وتم إجراء اختبار إليزا (الجيل الثالث) لكل

1

العينات والعينات الايجابية تم عمل اختبار رد فعل سلسلة البلمرة وكذلك الأجسام السطحية المضادة لفيروس بي الكبدي.

تنتهي الدراسة بالوصول إلى معدل انتشار وجود الأجسام المضادة لفيروس سي الكبدي بين النساء الحوامل وكذلك العوامل التنبؤية الموجودة لدى النساء الحوامل في المنطقة المذكورة.

وقد أظهرت الدراسة الأتي:

- من بين 360 سيدة حامل شاركن في الدراسة وجدنا 22 سيدة يحملن الأجسام المضادة لفيروس سي بالدم بنسبة 6.1% من إجمالي النساء المشاركات في البحث.

- وقد أظهرت الدراسة كذلك وجود علاقة ذات دلالة إحصائية بين وجود الأجسام المضادة لفيروس سي بالدم وبين العوامل التنبؤية التالية (ارتفاع سن السيدة الحامل وكذلك سن زوجها ووجود مرض كبدي سابق لدى الزوج).

ولم تتمكن الدراسة من إثبات علاقة ذات دلالة إحصائية بين وجود الأجسام المضادة لفيروس سي بالدم وبين العوامل التنبؤية التالية (عمليات جراحية سابقة- إجراءات طبية للأسنان- نقل دم- وشم- ختان- أدوية وريدية- زوج حامل للفيروس- تاريخ مرضي للفيروس داخل العائلة).

وبناء عليه نوصي بالتالي:

يتم عمل دراسة أخرى على السيدات الحوامل متضمنة عددا أكبر من السيدات للتعرف على أهم العوامل التنبؤية التي تؤدي الى وجود الأجسام المضادة لفيروس سي الكبدي بالدم.